DERMA*myth*

**CHESAHNA
KINDRED, MD,
MBA, FAAD**

DERMAmyth.

Dr. Sophia Red—
Thank you for being so
supportive. Congrats on your
growing family!
Dr. Kindred

TABLE OF CONTENTS

PART II HAIR CARE

PART III GENERAL

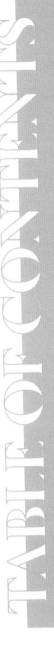

TABLE OF CONTENTS

Introducing   DERMA*myth*.

(I'm sure my colleagues will appreciate this.) When you come to the office, we (dermatologists) want to know what's wrong, how it's affecting you, and what helps or worsens the problem. We want to explain the diagnoses, treatment options, side effects, etc.

Unfortunately, time is wasted too often discussing myths. My contribution to the cause, **DERMA**myth.

Here we go!

SKIN

PART I

THE CONCERN IS NOT IF IT'S NATURAL OR UNNATURAL. THE CONCERN IS WHETHER IT'S TOXIC OR NON-TOXIC.

DR. KINDRED

DERMA*Myth*

NEOSPORIN

This DermaMyth covers Neosporin (if you listen carefully, you will hear the collective sighs of my fellow dermatologists). Neosporin is a widely used antibiotic ointment that dermatologist generally do not recommend for the following reasons:

- A wound that is not infected does not heal any better or faster by adding an antibiotic to petroleum jelly or Vaseline.

- One of the main ingredients in Neosporin, neomycin sulfate, was named Allergen of the Year in 2010. Neomycin is one of the major causes of allergic contact dermatitis aka allergic skin reactions. This means if you become allergic to neomycin from unnecessarily using Neosporin, your doctor would not be able to prescribe antibiotics in the same category as neomycin because of the allergy.

None of us feel that Neosporin is worth you going down that road. So, what do dermatologists (skin experts) recommend applying to simple wounds? Petroleum jelly (Vaseline, or Aquaphor if you want to be fancy). Please see a medical professional if you think you have an infected wound.

ONLY TEENS GET ACNE

Don't you wish acne magically disappeared for all of us by the age 21? About 40 to 50 million Americans suffer from acne. The myth that acne only afflicts teenagers is one that dermatologists and acne-sufferers alike wish would go away. According to the American Academy of Dermatology, there is a growing number of women with acne in their 30s, 40s, 50s, and beyond!

Women with acne tend to suffer from hormonal acne. One way to describe it, is the body becomes hypersensitive to its own testosterone. Effects include hormonal acne, facial hair, hair loss on the scalp, oily skin, sweating, irregular periods, and infertility. Studies show acne can cause low self-esteem, depression, dark spots on the skin, and permanent scars.

The good news is, acne isn't a mystery for board-certified dermatologists. Virtually, all acne will have a successful outcome with treatment. If you suffer from acne, please see a board-certified dermatologist.

DERMA*myth*

DIRTY CLIPPERS

Who hasn't heard the saying that dirty clippers cause ingrown hairs on the back of the scalp/neck? The medical term is Acne Keloidalis (aka Acne Keloidalis Nuchae, or AKN). AKN is inflammation of the hair follicle that is quickly followed by scars. The scars may turn into keloid-like growths.

Acne Keloidalis can be disfiguring and painful. It tends to affect black men more than other groups. Many believe that AKN is caused by "dirty clippers." Please, let's stop blaming our licensed barbers. Barbers typically use an antimicrobial solution that effectively kills the bacteria Staphylococcal Aureus (or Staph for short), the bacteria implicated in AKN.

Furthermore, AKN is also associated with friction against the back of the neck from tight collars and helmets; and trauma from shaving or short haircuts. For some reason, this condition is rarely seen in kids before puberty. If you suffer from AKN, please see a board-certified dermatologist.

EXTRA SUN EXPOSURE NATURALLY & SAFELY INCREASES VITAMIN D LEVELS

If this DermaMyth stops just one person from telling a dermatologist that "Sun exposure is a healthy way to reverse vitamin D deficiency/ low Vitamin D levels" then I would have added years to the dermatologist's life.

Facts:

- Vitamin D is critical to bone health.
- Sun exposure helps the body to make its own vitamin D.
- Sun exposure and especially indoor tanning are known to cause skin cancer, including melanoma, which is the deadliest form of cancer.
- About 75% of skin cancer deaths are from melanoma.
- The incidence of melanoma has been rising at an alarming rate for over 30 years.

Evidence that vitamin D lowers the death rate from cancers are inconsistent.

The American Academy of Dermatology states, "Vitamin D can be safely and easily obtained from a healthy diet that includes foods naturally rich in Vitamin D, food beverages fortified with vitamin D, and / or vitamin D supplements." So please, support your local dermatologist by not spreading the myth that the healthy way to increase your Vitamin D level is to increase sun exposure. Simply eat Vitamin D-rich foods such as salmon and mushrooms.

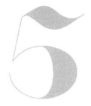
INDOOR TANNING IS SAFE

I still have patients who are convinced that indoor tanning is safe. Nope nope nope. Unless you're referring to a spray tan, indoor tanning is absolutely not safe. The W.H.O (World Health Organization) labels tanning beds as a carcinogen (cancer-causing) practice.

The artificial lights of the tanning beds emit the same amount of ultraviolet radiation as the sun- sometimes more! Studies show that the use of a tanning bed before the age of 35 increases the risk of melanoma by 75%. Melanoma is the deadliest form of skin cancer.

There is a trend of going to a tanning salon in preparation for summer. Even worse, some parents allow their children to frequent tanning salons in preparation for prom. It simply is not worth it. Your future self is thanking you now for never visiting a tanning bed again.

DERMA*Myth*

CHEMICAL-FREE SUNSCREEN AREN'T CHEMICALS

This DermaMyth covers the myth that physical sunscreens are chemical-free. Truthfully, all sunscreen ingredients are chemicals. Let's first discuss "chemical" vs "physical" sunscreens.

The physical sunscreens contain zinc and/or titanium. They physically block the ultraviolet rays from damaging the skin, like a shield. The chemical sunscreens usually contain avobenzone and oxybenzone, ingredients that use a chemical reaction to neutralize and absorb the ultraviolet rays like a sponge. Both protect your skin. Dr. Elizabeth Buzney, a board-certified dermatologist in Boston, points out that a more accurate classification system is whether or not the sunscreen ingredients are organic or inorganic.

Organic ingredients are carbon-based and include avobenzone and oxybenzone. Inorganic ingredients are zinc oxide and titanium oxide. So, while none of the sunscreens are "chemical-free," they are safe and very effective in reducing the signs of aging and development of skin cancers. If you have sensitive skin, you may prefer the physical sunscreens. If you have a melanin-rich skin tone, consider the chemical sunscreens to avoid a white residue.

DERMA*Myth*

COCOA BUTTER FOR STRETCH MARKS

The DermaMyth about cocoa butter and stretch marks go together like peanut butter and jelly. Whether or not you develop stretch marks is by far more related to your genes than how well you moisturize your skin. If you have dry skin, then go for it, as cocoa butter is a great moisturizer!

However, no cream can prevent stretch marks. Board-certified dermatologists often treat stretch marks with products containing retinoids or alpha hydroxy acids and sometimes lasers. The best time to start treating stretch marks is as early as possible.

DERMA*Myth*

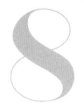

ACNE SCRUBBING BEADS

This DermaMyth focuses on the myth that if you scrub your acne, the acne will clear quicker. This is likely the trigger for tons of acne cleansers containing scrubbing beads on the market. Many of my colleagues will agree that scrubbing beads can often cause irritation that makes the dark marks or redness caused by acne to appear worse.

It is usually the other ingredients in the skin products and not the scrubbing beads that are most effective. So, save the environment and the fish in the sea by avoiding facial cleansers that contain scrubbing beads.

LARGE PORES

This DermaMyth covers large pores. Large pore size is a condition drowning in myths, particularly: Sun exposure shrinks pore size. Not true. The sun breaks down the collagen that keeps the pores tight.

For this reason, some board-certified dermatologists prescribe tretinoin to treat this condition. Enlarged pores are mostly genetic and worsened by excess oil production that clogs pores or exacerbated by small hairs that worsen the opening. Things that do work: tretinoin, chemical peel, laser, nose strips, and a few others. Please see your local board-certified dermatologist for treatment options best for you.

COCONUT OIL IS A GOOD SUNSCREEN

Just nope.

Criteria to look for in a sunscreen include:

- Broad Spectrum
- Water Resistant
- SPF 30 or higher
- Antioxidants

DON'T NEED SUN PROTECTION ON CLOUDY DAYS

This DermaMyth covers the myth that you don't need sun protection on cloudy days. The truth is, clouds block visible light (like light from a light bulb) but not harmful ultraviolet radiation that damage the skin.

In general, wear your facial moisturizer with sunscreen (spf 30+, broad spectrum, water resistant, antioxidants), sun glasses, hats, etc., as you would on a sunny day.

BENADRYL CREAM

This DermaMyth covers Benadryl or diphenhydramine. If you have an itchy rash, such as eczema or poison ivy, then by all means, take Benadryl, but only by mouth!

When you apply Benadryl cream to skin that is not intact, the Benadryl penetrates to the deeper layers of the skin and triggers an allergic reaction. Your local board-certified dermatologist kindly recommends that you take Benadryl by mouth when needed, but always avoid Benadryl cream.

BABY PRODUCTS

This DermaMyth covers "baby products." Very rarely does a board-certified dermatologist recommend "baby products" scented with that familiar heart-warming baby smell. These products are typically loaded with fragrances, preservatives, and allergens. With babies, simple is best. Regular old petroleum jelly is a dermatologist's best friend.

MELANOMA IS A WHITE DISEASE

This DermaMyth Monday covers the myth that melanoma, the deadly skin cancer, only occurs in white people and not black people. The myth probably draws from the fact that melanoma affects whites much more often than blacks. However, the myth is dangerous because when a black person does develop melanoma, the melanoma is more likely to kill that person than a white person.

Blacks tend to develop more aggressive types of melanomas. Furthermore, blacks are less likely to be diagnosed at an early stage in the disease process. As a result, an aggressive melanoma allowed to fester coupled with the myth that only whites develop melanoma is a deadly formula.

If you, regardless of your race, have a funny looking mole, a mole that suddenly changes in shape or size, or a mole that bleeds, please see a local board-certified dermatologist for an evaluation. More information is available at www.aad.com or www.spotskincarcer.org.

BLACK HENNA

This DermaMyth covers the myth that "black henna" is natural. Henna is derived from plant life native to Africa and southern Asia and leaves a red-brown stain. However, the chemical PPD or para-phenylenediamine is often added to henna, giving it a black color.

PPD is added to hair dyes and textile dyes; used as a photographic developing solvent; and more. Allergy to authentic henna is rare, but allergy to PPD is common. If you develop a rash to henna that is black and not red-brown, don't blame the henna! And, see your local board-certified dermatologist for appropriate treatment.

KELOIDS

This DermaMyth covers keloids. Specifically that stretching the scar will prevent a keloid from developing. While we have a lot to learn about the formation of keloids, we certainly know that tension on the scar is one of the triggers.

In fact, constant pressure flattens and weakens keloids. Keloid can be relentless. Keloids that are painful, tender, or itch are more likely to enlarge without treatment. If you have an active keloid, please see your local board-certified dermatologist for prompt treatment.

BANANA PEELS CURE WARTS

This DermaMyth covers the myth that banana peels cure warts. I can picture my dermatology colleagues doing the happy dance that I covered this myth. Home remedies that don't work for warts are as common as the warts themselves. Warts are caused by the virus in human papillomavirus (HPV). Sometimes, out of the blue, the immune system kicks in and decides to kill the virus, then the wart vanishes. This makes patients think that whatever treatment they used at the time was the cure.

"Treatments" I've heard patients tell me include: rubbing a raw potato on the wart on a full moon, garlic paste, banana peels, and the new fave, apple cider vinegar. I will admit, 3M silver ductape actually works. If you have a wart that doesn't improve with wart treatment products from the store, please see your local board-certified dermatologist.

TOOTHPASTE FOR PIMPLES

This DermaMyth covers using toothpaste to treat acne. The ingredients to form a pimple are clogged pores, dead skin, oil and bacteria. Toothpaste typically contain hydrogen peroxide, alcohol and triclosan, all ingredients that kill bacteria. This is the reason why some people notice a difference when they apply toothpaste to their pimples.

Bacteria fighting ingredients in a toothpaste makes sense because bacteria in the mouth release chemicals that break down the teeth and cause cavities. However, toothpaste was designed for teeth, not the skin. The redness, irritation, peeling and dark spots left on the skin caused by toothpaste often isn't worth it. There are much better and more effective ways to treat your acne. Please see a board-certified dermatologist for your acne.

MEDERMA FOR SCARS

This DermaMyth covers Mederma. Dermatologists really looked forward to Mederma when it originally came out over 10 years ago. Scientific study after study concluded that Mederma improved the appearance of scars. We soon realized that our patients were not seeing the benefit we expected.

Then, a study showed that Mederma did not work better than a dermatologist's favorite product: petroleum jelly. Add on the high cost of Mederma... you will rarely hear a board-certified dermatologist recommend Mederma over grandma's petroleum jelly.

BUTTER ON A BURN

This DermaMyth covers the myth advising you to apply butter to a burn. Applying non-sterile proteins on burns does not help. For 2nd and 3rd degree burns (the skin is blistering, is white, or has no feeling), you need to be treated by a physician. For 1st degree burns (skin is red but has a normal feeling) you usually can treat at home. Cool a minor burn by running cool water on it immediately. Apply petroleum jelly twice a day until healed.

MAKEUP AGES YOUR SKIN

This DermaMyth covers the myth that wearing makeup regularly ages your skin. More accurately, not REMOVING makeup at the end of each day (along with the build up of toxins from the day) damages skin cells. Damaged skin cells lead to discoloration and wrinkles, i.e., signs of aging.

Conversely, the sunscreen and antioxidants added to makeup makes makeup helpful. Visit your local board-certified dermatologist for advice about the best products outside of makeup that reverse the signs of aging. Your future self will thank you.

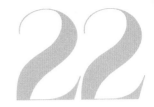
ALOE VERA

This DermaMyth covers aloe vera. Aloe vera has very useful properties. Some clearly over-exaggerate the benefits of aloe vera despite it being an otherwise great plant. Let's start with the great properties of aloe vera. Aloe vera has been used for medicinal purposes for millenia. Queens Nefertiti and Cleopatra used aloe vera as a part of their beauty regimens. Aloe vera contains several vitamins (a, c, e, B12, and folic acid); enzymes that reduce inflammation; minerals (calcium, copper, selenium, potassium, and zinc); anthraquinones that relieve pain, kill bacteria and viruses; and hormones that aid in wound healing.

Regarding wound healing (please forgive me if I get to nerdy), aloe vera increases collagen type III that leads to wound contraction and increases the strength of the scar tissue. Aloe vera also increases the concentration of the chemicals hyaluronic acid and dermatan sulfates, which are key players in wound healing. One of the worst consequences of wounds are infections. Aloe vera has anti-microbial effects, killing fungi, bacteria, and viruses. With these properties, there was no way aloe vera would rise untarnished by myths.

ALOE VERA

Continued

One myth is at aloe vera is safe. Everything that's natural isn't safe. Aloe vera can cause temporary redness and burning sensation but also full-blown allergic reactions. For those who ingest aloe: pregnant women must avoid eating aloe because aloe vera can cause uterine contractions. Breastfeeding women should avoid eating aloe because it may cause the baby's stomach to become upset. Patients with heart disease and diabetes should avoid ingesting aloe vera because it interacts with important and life-saving medications.

The 2nd popular myth about aloe vera is regarding sunburns. Aloe vera is like a Band-Aid to minor sunburns and can provide a soothing or cooling sensation, but doesn't prevent sunburns.

DERMA*Myth* 23

UROTHERAPY FOR ANTI-AGING

This DermaMyth covers the myth that urotherapy reverses the signs of aging in the skin. Urotherapy, or urine therapy, refers to the various applications using human urine for medicinal purposes. The theory is that your urine reverses the signs of aging. First of all, it's urine. Secondly, urine is mostly water with a small amount of urea. Urine is a WASTE PRODUCT!

The more hygienic and effective way to use urea is to purchase a urea lotion. There are over-the-counter and prescription strength urea medications. Urea helps with dry skin, eczema, psoriasis, and dry heels. If you have one of these conditions not controlled with over-the-counter medications, please consider seeing a local board-certified dermatologist before resorting to urine. Regarding the effect of aging, wrinkles, loss of collagen, deep wrinkles, and discoloration, go straight to your local dermatologist.

DERMA*Myth* **24**

ACNE AND MAKEUP

This DermaMyth covers the myth that you cannot wear makeup if you have acne. I can't tell you how often I am caught in the middle of a tense debate between a teenage girl and her parent about this issue! I try to be neutral, but my teenage patient is usually the one left smiling. The key to wearing makeup and not worsening your acne is to not clog your pores with products.

Be sure the label on your makeup says: won't clog pores, oil-free, non-comedogenic or non-acnegenic. Remember to remove the makeup daily, wash makeup brushes at least weekly and do not share makeup! I recommend loose mineral-based powder foundations. In the end, the patient wins the debate and may continue to wear makeup so long as the teen follows these guidelines. As always, if you have acne that doesn't improve despite these measures, please see your local board-certified dermatologist

USING FACE TOWELS

This DermaMyth covers the myth that you should wash your face with a washcloth. Yes, that's how many of us were raised, but hear me out. Unless you use a new face towel daily, your towel is very dirty. When you wash your face, you transfer germs and dead skin to the towel.

A damp towel is a breeding ground for germs: water, warm temperature, oxygen, food (your dead skin), and a neutral pH. The droplets from your toilet join the party when you flush since the face towel is stored in the bathroom. It is best to simply use clean hands to wash your face.

SKIN & HAIR PRODUCT LABELS

This DermaMyth covers the myth that products labeled, "#1 Dermatologist Recommended" or "Voted #1 by Dermatologists" mean that dermatologist everywhere vouch for this product. Yes, the labels imply we all vouch for the product, but this is often not the case.

Years ago, I attended one of the largest meetings for dermatologists. At this meeting, we learned about products directly from the skin care companies, including the chemists, researchers, etc.

A gigantic skin care company had a booth requesting dermatologists to complete a survey: Which gentle cleanser would you recommend to patients?

A. Ajax
B. Clorox bleach
C. (this company's gentle cleanser I won't name)
D. (A competitor's harsh antibacterial soap I won't name.)

Clearly, by far the majority of us incredulously asked if the survey was real because the options, except the company's own product, were absurd. We responded that if those were the only options, then of course C. And there you go, folks. That company could continue to label its soap as the "#1 dermatologist recommended gentle cleanser." The benefit of seeing your local board-certified dermatologist is that she/he can tell you the best products for your skin type and condition.

SLIME

This DermaMyth covers the myth that homemade slime is safe since it is made from household items. Last year my daughter made about a dozen different types of slime. How about yours?

Glitter slime, butter slime, neon slime, etc. Thankfully she avoided a reaction called contact dermatitis. Many people are becoming allergic to an ingredient in school glue called methylchloroisothiazolinone/ methylisothiazolinone (MCI/MI).

Others develop an irritation called irritant contact dermatitis to Borax. So, if your little scientist suddenly develops an itchy rash on the hands, the slime may be the culprit.

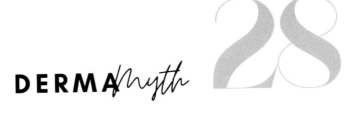
SONIC FACIAL BRUSH

This DermaMyth covers the myth that the sonic facial brushes worsen or cure acne. The brush is a tool, and is neither good or bad. The cleansing brushes are not necessary to cleanse your skin. My favorite is to use your clean hands. You may find the brushes are helpful to remove makeup. My favorite makeup removing strategy is to apply a moisturizer and gently wipe off with a tissue before washing your face.

The brush may enhance the effect of your topical medications. If you have heavy hands though, this could backfire. Do not SCRUB your face with the brush. Simply apply gentle pressure and let the sonic waves dislodge the dirt and debris from your skin. The "Clairsonic purge" occurs when someone experiences an outbreak soon after starting the brush. Often, this usually mirrors the "it worsens before it improves" phase. If you have sensitive skin, it may be best to consult your board-certified dermatologist first.

PART II

HAIR CARE

THERE ARE TONS OF PRODUCTS YOU CAN BUY FOR HAIR LOSS. THERE'S ONLY A FEW THAT ACTUALLY WORK.

DR. KINDRED

ONLY PAINFUL HAIR STYLING CAUSE TRACTION ALOPECIA

It's common knowledge that traction alopecia is caused by excessive tension that rips the hair follicle from the scalp. The tricky part is that hairstyles that lead to traction alopecia are NOT always painful. In this case, bumps (or traction folliculitis) develop a couple of days later.

Traction alopecia is common among ballerinas and gymnasts who chronically wear buns, those who wear tight braids and ponytail, and athletes who often wear headbands. If you notice tiny bumps along your hairline a couple of days after a new hair style, simply loosen or redo the hair in that area (ex. redo the braid, take down the pony tail, etc.).

TOO LATE TO TREAT ALOPECIA

This DermaMyth covers the myth that "it's too late to treat your hair loss." Yes, it is best to treat hair loss as early as possible. However, unless you are evaluated by a board-certified dermatologist who specializes in hair loss, don't give up!

BIOTIN

Evidence regarding biotin for hair loss overwhelmingly suggests that biotin does NOT reverse hair loss. (If you have hair loss, please see your local board-certified dermatologist with a niche in hair loss.) Biotin does help with nail growth, however. More importantly, "Biotin in blood or other samples taken from patients who are ingesting high levels of biotin in dietary supplements can cause clinically significant incorrect lab test results," the FDA says in a statement.

"The FDA has seen an increase in the number of reported adverse events, including one death, related to biotin interference with lab tests." Yes, taking biotin supplements can make your normal blood tests look abnormal and vice versa. At this time, I recommend my patients not to take biotin supplements for hair loss (never did really). Carefully check your hair supplements for high levels of biotin.

Source:
Patel DP, Swink SM, Castelo-Soccio L. A
Review of the use of biotin for hair loss. Skin Appendage Disord. 2017 Aug;3(3):166-169

CASTOR OIL

This DermaMyth is by special request: Overall, castor oil is not harmful. Castor oil is extracted from the seeds of the Ricinus communis (the castor bean) and used as emulsifying agents and surfactants in many skin/hair care products. Castor oil has been used in various rituals worldwide for millennia and is generally well tolerated with only a few cases of allergic contact dermatitis (allergic skin reaction) in the medical literature [source Toxicol Res 2015 June 3 (12); 105-136].

Thus, I see no issue with my patients applying castor oil to their hair. There is a case of a patient who applied castor oil and coconut oil and soon after trying to wash it out developed severe tangles resembling a bird's nest [Int J Trich. 2917 July-Sep;9 (3):116-118]. Not sure if the problem was the combination of the coconut oil and castor oil, just the coconut oil, or something the patient omitted from the story. At this time, there is zero, zilch, zip scientific evidence that castor oil reverses hair loss. If you suffer from hair loss, please see a board-certified dermatologist.

DANDRUFF MEANS YOU'RE NOT DRINKING WATER

This DermaMyth will save us all a lot of time. Dandruff, or seborrheic dermatitis, is caused by the yeast Malassezia, also known as Pityrosporum (keep in mind there are different types of yeast). It is the same yeast that causes cradle cap. Dermatologists generally treat the condition by killing the yeast (with shampoos, creams, or pills) and relieving the symptoms (itching, flaking, and scaling). Sometimes, the yeast will spread to the face mimicking dry skin or mimicking acne. Drinking water does not kill the yeast or reduce the symptoms. Now, if your sole reason for drinking water is because of dandruff, forget everything I said and drink up.

WEAVES = PROTECTIVE STYLE

This DermaMyth is dedicated to the myth that weaves = protective styles. Weaves are not "protective" simply because you're not combing or styling your own hair frequently. This is especially the case when the braids underneath the weave are so tight that they rip the hair follicle out of the scalp. This damage causes traction alopecia.

Furthermore, many do not wash their hair regularly enough when wearing a weave. If the braids are not too tight and the hair is washed on a regular basis, then by all means, weave away! But if you wear a weave, please keep this point in mind.

SHAVING HAIR MAKES IT GROW THICKER

How many times have you been told, "shaving will make you hair grow back thicker"? I wish it were true! With all of the patients with hair loss, I would hire a barber to sit outside my office and shave heads as patients walk in! I would set up a drive thru where patients lean their head out the car window while we shave scalps in an assembly line.

If this strategy worked, then our eyebrows would never thin as we age since ladies shape/shave/wax/pluck eyebrows regularly, over years! This would save us from biopsies, shampoos, pills, injections, and the myriad of other treatments required for alopecia. Alas, there is no biological basis about shaving the hair strand that tells the follicle to enlarge and grow more hair.

BRUSHING YOUR HAIR MAKES IT GROW

This DermaMyth covers that old wives' tale that brushing your hair a hundred strokes a day will help the hair to grow. Nope! It will help your hair to grow on your brush because brushing beyond detangling or styling only makes you prone to hair breakage. Brushing the hair too hard can also rip the follicle out of the scalp, causing traction alopecia.

HAIR TRANSPLANTATION CURES HAIR LOSS

This DermaMyth covers hair transplantation. Hair transplantation is essentially borrowing from Peter to pay Paul. Hair is removed from the root in one section of the scalp (usually the back) and placed in the area of hair loss. Most forms of hair loss are relentless (androgenetic alopecia, female pattern baldness, male pattern baldness, central centrifugal cicatricial alopecia, frontal fibrosing alopecia, or temporary alopecia areata, traction alopecia, etc.).

Rarely does a patient have a form of hair loss that hair transplantation CURES, such as severe permanent traction alopecia. Long term management should be expected. Board-certified dermatologists want you to remember that medical treatment is essential.

HEAD LICE

This DermaMyth covers head lice. One myth is that head lice affects people with dirty hair, which is not true. In fact, head lice could not care less whether the hair is clean or dirty as they're looking for human blood to survive. Each year, 6-12 million children between the ages of 3 and 12 years old get head lice. About 10% of caucasian children get head lice each year compared to only 0.3% of black children. This leads us to the other myth that blacks do not get head lice. The nits or eggs must adhere to the hair strands, but the use of hair oils in black culture makes the hair strand too slippery and straightening treatments such as flat irons and hot combs kill the lice.

Another reason why there's a low incidence of lice in black people is that head lice have adapted to hold onto hair strands with a round shape while the hair of black people is an oval shape. Hair styling practices brings us to the next myth: hair color does not kill lice. In fact, neither does hairspray or hair gels. Yes, there are several myths surrounding head lice. Board-certified dermatologists usually are not required for treatment as the over-the-counter remedies are effective (permethrin). However, if you have trouble getting rid of the lice, or if you develop and infection from scratching, you should see a board-certified dermatologist.

SCALP MASSAGES

This DermaMyth covers the myth that scalp massages reverse hair loss. The reasoning I've come across is that scalp massages increase the flow of blood to the scalp, flooding the hair follicles with oxygen and nutrients and thereby overpowering the diseases that lead to hair loss. As a result, the hair grows. The truth is, because the scalp is so close to the brain, there is quite a rich blood flow to scalp.

There is no scientific evidence that increasing blood flow to the already well-vascularized scalp reverses hair loss. Now, if scalp massages reduce your stress level, feels great to you or relaxes you, by all means, massage away. It is not harmful.

GREASE YOUR SCALP DAILY

This DermaMyth covers the myth about greasing the scalp. It is a common belief that one should apply hair grease to the scalp on a regular basis. The benefits are that it camouflages flaking and relieves itching. In the winter, the skin produces more oil (sebum) to combat dryness. The yeast Malassezia, also known as Pityrosporum, thrives on sebum. The skin reacts to the high yeast count with itching, flaking, and even bumps that mimic acne when yeast spreads to the face. Instead of camouflaging the symptoms, dermatologists recommend getting to the root of the problem: kill the yeast. At home, use anti-dandruff shampoos (avoid onces that make the hair dry and brittle) or, add a few drops of tea tree oil to your favorite shampoo. Hydrocortisone helps relieve itching and flaking. If these measures don't work, please see your local board-certified dermatologist.

RICE WATER

This DermaMyth covers the myth that rice water reverses hair loss. I first heard of this a couple of years ago and thought it would die out. However, this myth is still trending. Le sigh...

First, rice water is made by soaking rice in water for several hours. After removing the rice, the leftover water is used to soak the hair. My reason for advising my patients against this practice: that is exactly one of the methods for removing arsenic from rice! But instead, you are soaking your hair with the arsenic-containing rice water!

Quick discussion about arsenic. Arsenic is an element in the Earth's crust, and is naturally present in water, air, and soil. It develops naturally in the environment and as a result of arsenic-containing pesticides. Because arsenic is naturally found in the soil and water, it is absorbed by plants regardless of whether the plants are grown organically or not.

RICE WATER

Continued,

In other words, organic rice has just as much arsenic as regular rice. Long-term exposure to high levels of arsenic is associated with higher rates of skin, bladder and lung cancers, as well as heart disease. Arsenic poisoning occurs with ingestion.

While rice water has some nutrients (thiamine and niacin), rice is actually nutrition-poor to begin with. To nourish the hair, it's best to use conditioning products designed for the hair. If you have hair loss, instead of soaking your hair in an arsenic solution, please see a board-certified dermatologist. By the way, reports say the best technique to remove arsenic is to soak the rice in water overnight and discard the water, then cook the rice in a 5:1 water-to-rice ratio (like pasta).

VITAMIN E FOR HAIR LOSS

This DermaMyth covers the myth that applying Vitamin E to the scalp reverses hair thinning. I chose this topic because I've suddenly seen a lot of people promoting the application of Vitamin E directly to the scalp. Vitamin E is a great antioxidant. I heard of applying Vitamin E to wounds and other ailments since I was a child. The connection to hair loss is likely from a small study of less than 40 people: those that consumed Vitamin E grew longer hair than those that consumed a placebo (sugar pill) over several months. It was not applied to the scalp.

So, let's first talk about taking Vitamin E supplements. Over-supplementation of certain nutrients, including selenium, Vitamin A, and Vitamin E, has actually been linked to hair loss. Only 15 mg a day is recommended and your primary doctor and I both recommend avoiding excess intake of Vitamin E. The effects of high Vitamin E levels in your system include bleeding and decrease thyroid hormone production. Vitamin E even interferes with medications, including chemotherapy medications.

VITAMIN E FOR HAIR LOSS

Continued,

Vitamin E is regularly found in green leafy vegetables and fortified cereals. To increase intake of Vitamin E, people can eat foods that are naturally rich in this Vitamin. Some good food sources of Vitamin E include:

1 tablespoon of wheat germ oil – 20.3 mg
1 ounce (oz) of dry roasted sunflower seeds – 7.4 mg
1 oz of dry roasted almonds – 6.8 mg
2 tablespoons of peanut butter – 2.9 mg
Half a cup of boiled spinach – 1.9 mg
Half a cup of boiled broccoli – 1.2 mg

Experts generally consider increasing the intake of foods that contain Vitamin E to be safe. There is no robust evidence that applying Vitamin E to scalp will make the hair grow.

RELAXERS CAUSE CCCA

This DermaMyth covers the myth that relaxers cause Central Centrifugal Cicatricial Alopecia or CCCA. CCCA is the most common form of hair loss in black women. If you add the total number of black women suffering from the other 15 or so forms of hair loss, it still does not add up to the number of black women suffering from CCCA alone. This is the basis of myths that even dermatologists have spread. We have said that hot combs caused CCCA (previously called "Hot Comb Alopecia"). Then we blamed relaxers. Then we blamed braids. From experience with patients, I have long believed that these hair care practices can worsen CCCA, but not cause it.

There are amazing people making breakthroughs in this field. Through research, dermatologists have confirmed our suspicions that the disease is inherited and uncovered the fact that genes related to scarring are active in CCCA. For the most recent groundbreaking news, researchers may have found THE GENE for CCCA, PAD13. Are you as excited as I am? Forgive me for getting too nerdy, but I want to break this down in a way for non-medical people to understand (as I do in the office).

RELAXERS CAUSE CCCA

Continued..

Genes are blueprints or codes for proteins. The PADI3 gene encodes an enzyme. Enzymes are proteins that make reactions happen better or faster. PADI3 is the blueprint for the enzyme "peptidyl arginine deiminase, type III." This enzyme is responsible for shaping the proteins that form the hair. Patients with CCCA were found to have genes with errors, which leads to problem after problem in the hair production process (proteins in the wrong side of the cell, not enough of the enzymes available, proteins folded into the wrong shape, etc.).

You now have a bad product; the immune system's job is to rid your body of bad products (such as cancer cells, infections, etc). As a result, your body thinks the immune system is doing the right thing in getting rid of the hair. The immune system destroys the hair by flooding the scalp with inflammation. The end result is CCCA. Thank you to all the researchers that help me take better care of my patients!

JADE ROLLERS

This DermaMyth covers the myth that jade rollers reverse the sign of aging. Jade rollers are affordable beauty devices used for centuries in China but have recently become trendy in the US. It consists of a handle with a roller made of jade on one or both ends. Of course, as with other trends, jade rollers have been given magical properties beyond what is realistic. Some claim that jade rollers reverse wrinkles, minimize pores, and have anti-aging properties. Now let's look at the true effects of jade rollers.

One benefit is that jade does not harbor bacteria and other germs. If you recall the previous DermaMyth, we no longer use wash cloths for our face for this reason. You may use the jade roller instead of your fingers to gently rub in lotions and serums. Have you heard of using a cool spoon to remove eye puffiness when you wake up? In the same way that you would ice a swollen joint to reduce the swelling and inflammation, you may do so with a cold jade roller by storing it in the fridge. Here, the cool temperature is the key. You could do the same thing with a cold spoon. If you don't have a board-certified dermatologist, then you may appreciate these subtle benefits of a jade roller. However, if you do, please do not expect the same level of results as our in-office treatments: evaluation/ education, prescriptions, medical-grade serums, chemical peels, micro-needling, laser treatments, etc.

PART III

GENERAL

FOCUS ON THE
UNDERLYING PROBLEM
AND THE REST FALLS INTO
BALANCE.

DR. KINDRED

GLUTEN-FREE DIET

This DermaMyth covers the myth that gluten-free skin products are healthier than traditional skin products. Honestly, gluten-free skin products are a waste of money. Gluten is too large to absorb through the skin and can cause an allergic reaction.

People with a true gluten allergy develop digestive and skin problems from ingestion of gluten. Some may mistaken the skin symptoms to be the result of a skin product. When studied, exposure to gluten through the skin did not trigger a gluten allergy. If you have a gluten-free product that you love, no need to stop using it. However, if you are paying a premium for your gluten free products because someone convinced you it was healthier, save your money.

A study by the Mintel Group, "The Unintended Consequences of a Gluten-Free Diet" found that 25% of Americans report being on a gluten-free diet. In the article, the gluten-free group had higher levels of lead, mercury, cadmium, and arsenic than the group on a normal diet. Worse arsenic levels were more than just high, they were toxic! The suspected reason is that many gluten-free diets are rice-based. Rice is a natural source of arsenic. Reducing carbohydrate intake is not quite the same as avoiding gluten. Be healthy.

SNS NAILS

This DermaMyth covers the incredibly popular SNS or powder gel nails. Commonly, the nail technician will tell you that the powder gel nails are safe and healthy for your nails because they do not require ultraviolet radiation exposure. While this is true, keep in mind that the removal process damages your natural nail. The natural nail plate is thinned from the drill and acetone soaking dehydrates the nail plate. This leads to thinning, splitting, and peeling of the nail plate. If this has happened to you, applying petroleum jelly to your nails twice a day will help.

ALKALINE WATER

This DermaMyth covers the myths surrounding alkaline water. Alkaline water is less acidic than tap water. The water is typically treated by a machine that raises pH levels through a process called electrolysis. Pure water has a pH of about 7 while alkaline water has a pH > 7. Many bottled waters and tap water may have a pH < 7 , making it more acidic. The good thing about alkaline water is that it contains minerals sometimes such as calcium, potassium, and magnesium. There may be a specific population that benefits from alkaline water, but the research shows that the benefits stop there.

Our bodies do an incredible job of monitoring and controlling the ideal pH range required. Each organ system has its own unique pH range. An alkaline pH is not necessarily healthy. For example, an alkaline pH is sometimes the result of kidney disease. It is also known that alkaline water is not completely safe. When drinking alkaline water, it contacts the small intestine, making it overly alkaline. This potentially leads to urinary tract infections, high blood pressure, anxiety, abnormal heartbeat, and more.

If your body cannot control your blood pH, before purchasing alkaline water, it is best to get to the underlying problem and find out why. I recommend discussing with your primary care physician before drinking alkaline water regularly.

PARABENS

This DermaMyth covers Parabens. Parabens are a group of preservatives added to personal care products such as deodorant, shampoos, and even toothpaste, to stop the growth of harmful mold, fungi and bacteria. These individual products carry low or even "safe" amounts of parabens.

However, since 90% of common items found in grocery stores contain parabens, the concentration in our bloodstream adds up. Herein lies the controversy: do parabens cause cancer or not? If so, what amount of parabens leads to cancer?

Parabens are suspected endocrine-disrupting chemicals, meaning they mimic hormones in our body. The body then has to decide whether or not to treat the paraben as a hormone. Some believe that the body sometimes treat parabens as estrogen, triggering a chain reaction that can led to breast cancer. This is not yet proven. Beyond what's written here, there is a lot more hearsay and gossip. For now, the Kindred Hair & Skin Center products, such as our sunscreens, are paraben-free.

DERMA*Myth* 49

PROVIDER=DOCTOR

This DermaMyth covers the myth that it is okay to call your doctor a "provider." Calling your doctor a provider is a professional insult. Dr. Niran Al-Agba, a pediatrician in Washington state, wrote an article educating me on the origin of using the term "provider" in place of "doctor" or "physician." It turns out the origin of the term is more atrocious than I imagined. The term "provider" was first used by the Third Reich, yes, the Nazis – to belittle and systematically humiliate Jewish doctors as medical professionals. No further explanation necessary.

DERMA*Myth* 50

CROSSING YOUR LEGS CAUSES VARICOSE VEINS

This DermaMyth covers the myth that crossing your legs causes varicose veins. The most likely reason one has varicose veins is because it runs in the family. If you smoke, quit. Smoking is a risk factor for varicose veins ; as is pregnancy, lack of physical activity, inactivity, high blood pressure, and obesity.

Hair stylists and other occupations that require long periods of standing are also at risk. While avoiding crossing your legs doesn't improve or prevent varicose veins, you may notice improvement with leg elevations and compression stockings. Many dermatologists offer laser treatment for varicose veins but also refer patients to vascular surgeons when necessary.

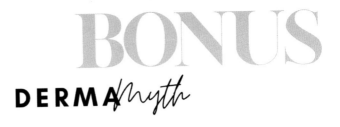

SKIN EXPERTS

This DermaMyth covers the myth that "skin expert" = dermatologist. The true experts are in fact Board-Certified Dermatologists. Those who fall short of earning this title get away with using other terms such as skin expert, skin doctor, skin specialist, one with a passion for skin, a holistic approach to skin, a board-certified physician specializing in skin, and the list goes on. Board-certified dermatologists complete (after college):

4 years of medical school
1 year internship in internal medicine, pediatrics or general surgery
3 years of an accredited dermatology residency
12,000 – 16,000 hours of patient care, and
Certification through the American Board of Dermatology or the American Osteopathic Board of Dermatology.

Anything short of this, is not a board-certified dermatologist. Beware of the fake dermatologists.

ANYTIME THE BODY IS THE PROBLEM, THERE IS NO CURE.

DR. KINDRED

About the Author

Dr. Chesahna Kindred is a board-certified dermatologist, published research author, and national speaker. She grew up in South Central, Los Angeles, an area of California known for its tough streets and strong community spirit, and a place where overcoming adversity was not simply a choice, but a way of life. It was this environment that planted the seed for Dr. Kindred's future in her field, cultivating a strong ambition and drive to serve her community, empowering people through beauty.

Growing up she quickly garnered a reputation for her love of education and her desire to help others achieve their goals. It was this drive that led her to pursue a career within the field of dermatology. Dr. Kindred began her studies at the University of Southern California where she received her Bachelor of Science with a minor in Spanish. She then relocated to Ohio where she continued to push herself in her educational pursuits, earning not just her MD degree, but also an MBA at the University of Cincinnati.

Dr. Kindred was awarded a full scholarship as a Yates Fellow for the MBA program, where she was only the third person in the history of the University of Cincinnati to receive the dual MD/MBA degree. She then took up her residency and fellowship at Howard University, an institution that pioneered Ethnic Dermatology. It was here that Dr. Kindred gained her passion and focus on hair loss and ethnic skin.

Soon after graduating from her dermatology residency at Howard University, she became a leading dermatologist at MedStar Health in the Baltimore area. Five years later, she founded Kindred Hair & Skin Center in Columbia, Maryland where she treats people of all ages and ethnicities. Her office is the first dermatology office worldwide with a full-service salon that specializes in hair loss.

About the Author (continued)

Locally, Dr. Kindred is heavily involved in community service, often organizing health fairs, mentoring aspiring doctors, and working with local churches and community organizations to help educate and empower the community at large. Within the field of dermatology, Dr. Kindred is chair, founder, or member of several professional and community organizations.

Within the field of dermatology, Dr. Kindred is
Founder and President, Onyx Medical Society
Chair of the National Medical Association, Dermatology Section
Fellow of the American Academy of Dermatology (FAAD)
Member of the Women's Dermatological Society, American Society of Dermatologic Surgery, Maryland Dermatologic Society, and Monumental Dermatology Society

Outside of dermatology, Dr. Kindred is
Chair of the African American Community Roundtable, Health Committee
Leader of Celebration Church Health & Wellness Ministry
Deacon at Celebration Church at Columbia, Maryland

Dr. Kindred has several publications concerning an array of dermatologic topics including co-writing chapters in leading dermatology textbooks. Her publications include, but are not limited to, hair loss, skin cancer, and treatments in patients with skin of color. Philosophically, her focus of "Empowering through beauty" has resonated with patients worldwide. Understanding the desire people have to feel as beautiful outside as they do within, Dr. Kindred helps them achieve the balance that allows people to feel complete. True beauty is not about vanity, but instead about empowering one's self to have the confidence to live life to the fullest. Dr. Kindred resides in Maryland with her husband and two beautiful children.

Dedication
&
Acknowledgements

Dedication

This book is dedicated to my family and my village.

I come from a line of Grand Midwives; I start with them and say, Thank you. Also to my great grandmother, Tempe Anne, who was enslaved in Mississippi. I hope I am the fruition of you all's wildest dreams. This is dedicated to both of my grandmothers, Elouise Kindred and Alice Haskell, neither of whom could attend school past the 8th and 5th grades, respectively, but was able to send their children to college. To my parents, Albert Kindred and Charlotte Haskell, you raised me to believe I could be anything even the US President one day, until the world convinced me otherwise. I will never let that happen again.

To my sisters, for reminding me that I was a role model. Of course, to my children, Machela and Kingston, I hope I never let the world convince you that you cannot be anything you want to be. Most obviously, to my husband, for putting up with my activism, community service, leadership roles and now a book! You remain our protector, planner, and leader. Now most of all, this book is dedicated to God, who has always clearly answered my special prayer, "Jesus, please make the choice you want for me blatantly obvious."

This book is dedicated to my villages. My church village, natural hair stylist village, community service village, race equity work village, dermatology village, Howard University village, NMA village, troop village, mentee/mentor village, patient village, and more. If I left out anyone, please blame it on my mind and not my heart.

Acknowledgements

I would like to thank everyone who helped with this book:

My sister, Terica Kindred, for planting the seed.

Sierra Arnold of Madison Public Relations, for making it stylish, staying on fire, and unselfishly paying attention to every detail whether it was your lane or not.

Staff at Kindred Hair & Skin Center, for being amazing.

Scores of patients that provide fodder for this book, especially the patient that said to me with a straight face,
"But the internet said..."

Whitney Hogans, for giving me that push.

Kevin Bullock, my photographer.

Thank You,

Dr. Kindred

NOTES

NOTES

Made in the USA
Middletown, DE
12 September 2020

18012790R00042